Mediterranean Recipe Collection

50 Amazing Mediterranean Recipes for Your Daily Healthy Meals

Jenna Violet

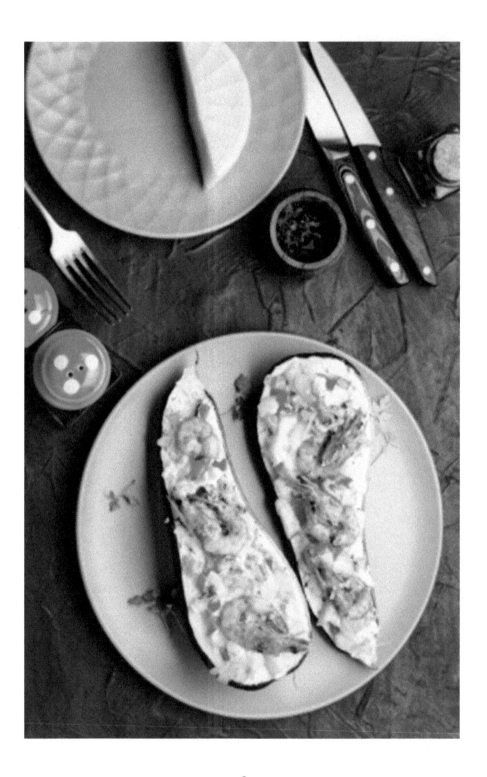

By reading this document, the reader agrees that under no circumstances is the author responsible for any losses, direct or indirect, which are incurred as a result of the use of information contained within this document, including, but not limited to, — errors, omissions, or inaccuracies.

Table of Contents

Quinoa tabbouleh

Ingredients

- ½ teaspoon pepper
- ½ teaspoon of salt
- ¼ cup of lemon juice
- 2 tablespoons of olive oil
- 1/3 cup of minced parsley
- 2 cups of water
- 1 can of black beans washed and drained; should be 15 ounces
- 1 cup of quinoa
- 1 small chopped sweet red pepper
- 1 small peeled and chopped cucumber

Directions

- Put water to boil in a large saucepan.
- Add the quinoa
- Reduce the heat to allow it to simmer and to absorb the extra liquid for 12 – 15 minutes.
- Remove the content from heat and fluff it with a fork.
- Transfer to another bowl to allow complete cooling.
- Introduce the cucumber, beans, parsley, and beans.
- In a small bowl whisk all the remaining ingredients, then drizzle over the salad and toss to coat.
- Refrigerate the content until it is chilled.

- Serve and enjoy

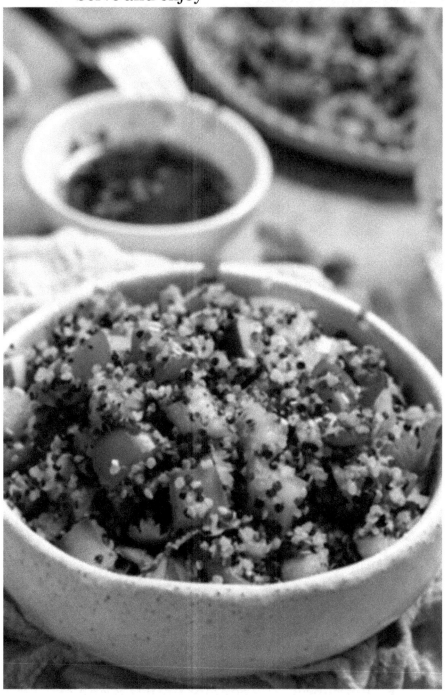

Parmesan chicken with artichoke hearts

Ingredients

- 2 thinly sliced green onions
- 4 boneless skinless chicken breast 6 ounces
- 1 lemon equally cut into 8 slices
- ¼ cup of shredded parmesan cheese
- 2 chopped garlic cloves
- 1 medium coarsely chopped onions
- 3 teaspoons olive oil
- ½ teaspoon of pepper
- 2 cans of water-packed artichokes hearts properly drained (should be 14 ounces each)
- ½ teaspoon of dried thyme
- 1 teaspoon of dried crushed rosemary
- ½ cup of white wine

Directions

- Begin by preheating the oven to 375°.
- Place the chicken in a baking pan with a thin coated cooking spray.
- Drizzle with 1 teaspoon of oil.
- Mix the rosemary, peppers, and thyme then sprinkle half of the mixture over the chicken.
- In a large bowl, combine onions, wine, garlic, artichokes hearts, remaining oil and mixture of herbs then toss to coat.
- Arrange the chicken and sprinkle with cheese then top with lemon slices.

- Roast the content until the thermometer reads 165° in 20 – 25 minutes.
- Evenly sprinkle with green onions
- Serve

Creamy feta-spinach dip

This recipe can turn out to be more addictive and powerful dip because of the garlic and feta ingredients. Do not worry, the addictiveness is due to the irresistibility delicious tasted the keep one hooked to continuously keep longing for more of it. The ingredients and directions are shown below.

Ingredients

- Fresh vegetables
- 1 teaspoon of dill weed
- 1/8 teaspoon of pepper
- 1 minced garlic glove
- 1 cup of chopped fresh spinach
- ¼ cup of less fat sour cream
- 1 cup of fatless plain yogurt
- 2 ounces of fatless cubed cream cheese
- ¾ cup of crumbled feta cheese

Directions

- Using a four layered cheesecloth, place is above a bowl.
- Put yogurt in the prepared four layered cheesecloth o strainer.
- Cover the edges of the yogurt with the cheesecloth.
- Keeping it under refrigeration for about 2 hours to a point when the yogurt has completely thickened in a uniform manner to the whipped cream.

- Transfer the yogurt to a food processor while the remaining liquid in the bowl can be discarded
- Introduce the feta cheese, sour cream, garlic, cream cheese then cover it until content has completely smoothened.
- Transfer to a small bowl where the spinach can then be stirred with the dill and pepper.
- Cover and refrigerate until when chilled.
- Serve with the vegetable and enjoy the taste.

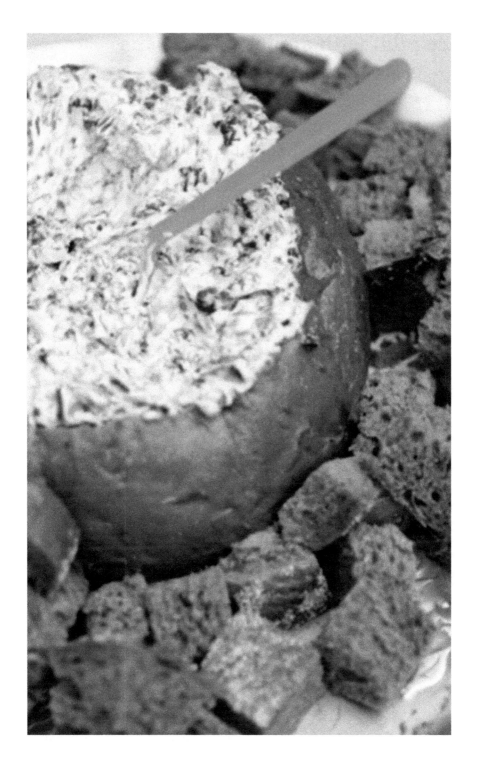

Rice pilaf with apples and raisins

Ingredients

- 1/8 teaspoon of cayenne pepper
- ¼ teaspoon of ground allspice
- ¼ teaspoon of dried thyme
- 1 teaspoon of salt
- ¼ teaspoon of ground cinnamon
- 1 cup of water
- 2 tablespoons of olive oil
- ¼ cup of golden raisin
- 1 cup of uncooked jasmine rice
- 1 small chopped onion
- ¼ cup of chopped apples

Directions

- Using a large saucepan, heat the oil over a medium temperature.
- Sauté onions until when they become tender in 4 – 6 minutes.
- Add the rice, then cook and stir until when the rice turns brown in about 4 – 6 minutes.
- Introduce in the remaining ingredients and bring to boil.
- Reduce the heat to allow it to simmer when covered to absorb the liquid until the rice is tender in 15 – 20 minutes.
- Fluff with a fork
- Serve

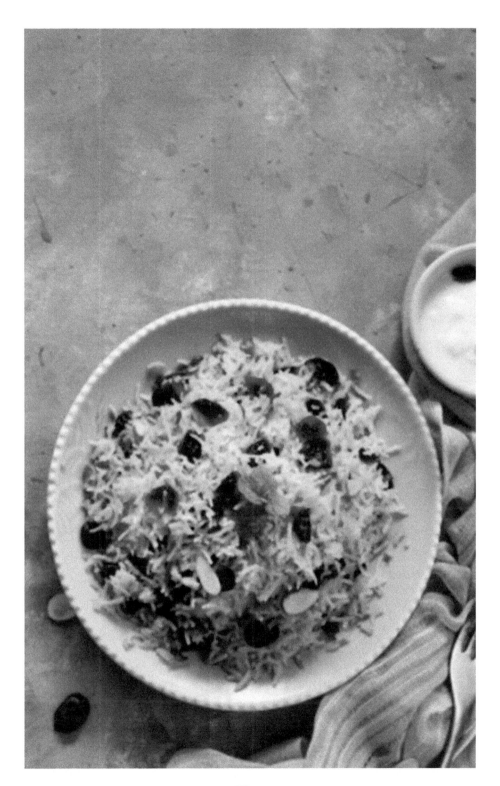

Mediterranean chicken

The preparation of this recipe is quite simple, yet heavy and irresistibly delicious in taste particularly when dressed with tomatoes, capers and olives. This is a real knockout dish for several individuals and families.

Ingredients

- 1 pint of grape tomatoes
- 3 tablespoons of drained capers
- ¼ teaspoon of salt
- 3 tablespoon of olive oil
- ¼ teaspoon of peppers
- 16 pitted ripe sliced Greek olives
- 4 boneless skinless chicken breast which should be approximately 6 ounces each when halved

Directions

- Ultimately, start the cooking by sprinkling the chicken with pepper and salt.
- In an ovenproof large skillet, cook in the oil over a medium temperature until when it turns to golden brown in about 2 – 3 minutes on every side.
- Add the capers, tomatoes, and olives.
- Bake while uncovered at about 475° until when the thermometer reading drops to 170° in 10 – 14 minutes.
- Serve and enjoy

Slim Greek deviled eggs

Only try out this recipe if you are ready to enjoy a finger licking delicious variation with deviled eggs. They are easy to make yet popular contribution to a brunch of tasty home kitchen.

Ingredients

- 1/8 teaspoon of pepper
- ½ teaspoon of grated lemon zest
- 1/8 teaspoon of salt
- ½ teaspoon of lemon juice
- 6 hard ready boiled large eggs
- 1 teaspoon of oregano
- 3 tablespoons of fatless mayonnaise
- 2 tablespoons of crumbled feta cheese
- Greek olives (optional)

Directions

- Lengthwise, cut the eggs into half.
- Completely remove the yolk and put aside the whites and the yolks.
- Using a large bowl, mash the reserved yolks.
- Stir in the mayonnaise, oregano, feta, lemon juice, lemon zest, pepper, and salt.
- Stuff into the egg whites.
- If desired, garnish with the Greek olives.
- Let it chill until ready to serve
- Enjoy

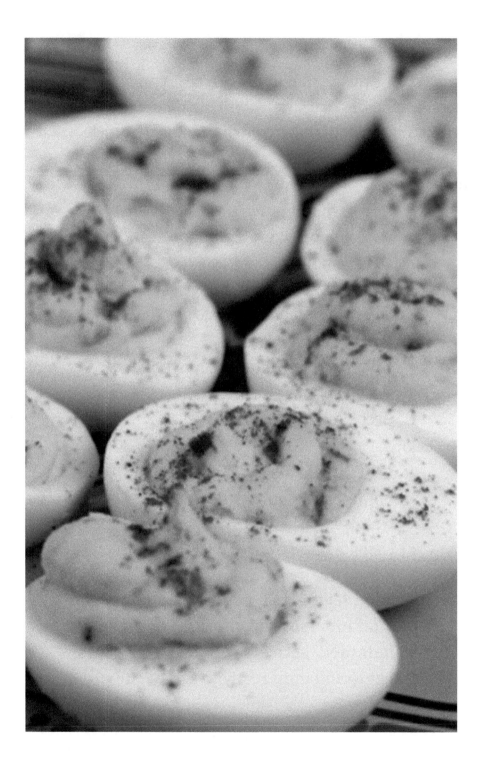

Greek tofu scramble

Ingredients

- 2 tablespoon of nutritional yeast
- juice of ½ lemon
- salt and pepper
- 1 tablespoon of oil
- ¼ small red onion, diced
- 2 cloves garlic, minced
- ½ cup of red bell pepper, diced
- 8 ounces of firm tofu
- 1 handful of fresh spinach
- ¼ cup of fresh basil, chopped
- ¼ teaspoon of salt
- ¼ cup of Kalamata olives, pitted and halved
- 11 teaspoon of tahini paste
- ½ cup of cherry tomatoes, halved

Directions

- In a small bowl, crumble tofu to the texture of scrambled eggs.
- Add nutritional yeast, tahini, lemon juice, and salt and keep aside.
- In a large skillet , heat oil over medium heat.
- Add onions and sauté for 5 minutes, stirring occasionally.
- Add bell pepper and garlic and sauté for another 5 minutes until the bell pepper is tender.

- Stir crumbled tofu and Kalamata olives.
- Heat all the way through, stirring occasionally.
- Add spinach and basil.
- Stir to wilted slightly, reducing to about half its size.
- Remove from heat and stir in cherry tomatoes.
- Season with salt and pepper.
- Serve and enjoy.

Greek veggie tacos

Ingredients

- 6 Kalamata olives
- 2 soft taco shells
- 2 tablespoons of crumbled feta cheese
- 2 tablespoons of hummus
- 2 tablespoons of Greek dressing
- 2 tablespoons of thinly sliced and chopped red onion
- 4 slices of cucumber, quartered
- 1 Roma tomato, cubed
- Leafy green lettuce

Directions

- Begin by spreading 1 tablespoon of hummus onto each soft taco.
- Fill tacos with cucumbers together with the tomatoes, red onions, olives and crumbled feta.
- Top with 1 tablespoon of Greek dressing on each.
- Serve and enjoy.

Kalamata olive spread

Ingredients

- ½ teaspoon of dried oregano
- ½ cup of pitted Kalamata olives
- 1 teaspoon of red wine vinegar

Directions

- Use an immersion blender, blend all ingredients together until smooth.
- Store in a sealed container in the refrigerator.
- Serve and enjoy.

Pan-seared citrus shrimp

Ingredients

- 1 medium lemon, cut into wedges
- 1 cup of fresh orange juice
- ½ cup of fresh lemon juice
- 5 garlic cloves, minced or pressed
- 3 pounds of medium shrimp, peeled and deveined
- 1 tablespoon of finely chopped red onion
- 1 tablespoon of olive oil
- 1 medium orange, cut into wedges
- Pinch of red pepper flakes
- Freshly ground black pepper and kosher salt
- 1 tablespoon of chopped fresh parsley

Directions

- In a medium bowl, whisk together the olive oil with orange juice, lemon juice, 2 teaspoons of the parsley, garlic, onion, and pinch of red pepper flakes.
- Pour the mixture into a large skillet set over medium heat.
- Bring to a simmer and cook until reduced by half in 8 minutes.
- Add the shrimp.
- Season with kosher salt and freshly ground black pepper.
- Cover let cook until they turn pink in 5 minutes.

- Top with the remaining parsley
- Serve and enjoy with orange and lemon slices on the side.

Hummus toast

Making hummus traditionally is a lot fun and tastier yet with no fuss and additional flavors. This recipe is simply a plain and classic recipe. Note, the outcome of the recipe should be thick, rich, smooth, and creamy.

Ingredients

- Hot water
- Sumac
- 3 to 4 ice cubes
- ⅓ cup tahini paste
- Early Harvest Greek extra virgin olive oil
- Juice of 1 lemon
- ½ teaspoon of kosher salt
- 3 cups cooked and peeled chickpeas
- 1 to 2 garlic cloves, minced

Directions

- In a bowl of a food processor, introduce the minced garlic together with the chickpeas.
- Start to puree until a visible smooth powder like mixture appears.
- Add the ice cubes, salt, lemon juice, and tahini while the processing is still running.
- Continue to blend for 4 minutes about.
- In the event that the thick semi-liquid solution is still too thick, add more water to dilute while the processor is still running.
- Blend until the solution turns silky smooth.

- Get a serving bowl, spread in it and then add early harvest extra virgin olive oil with drizzle.
- Add some chickpeas in the middle.
- Sprinkle the top with sumac
- Serve and enjoy with warm pita wedges and other veggies you like.

Foul mudamma recipe

This recipe simply involves stewing broad or fava beans which is seasoned with ground cumin finished with extra virgin olive oil. The Egyptians love to enjoy it with warm pita bread, fresh veggies, lemon juice and also herbs.

Ingredients

- Diced 1 tomato
- 1 large lemon juice
- Extra virgin olive oil
- ½ cup water
- 1 to 2 hot peppers, chopped
- 2 chopped garlic cloves
- Kosher salt
- 2 cans plain fava beans
- ½ to 1 teaspoon ground cumin
- 1 cup chopped parsley

To Serve

- Sliced cucumbers
- Olives
- Warm pit bread
- Green onions
- Sliced tomatoes

Directions

- In a saucepan, add ½ cup of water and the fava beans.
- Warm it over a medium temperature
- Season it with cumin and kosher salt.

- Mash the beans.
- Add hot peppers together with garlic in a mortar and pestle, then smash them.
- Introduce one lemon juice, stir to blend
- Over the fava beans, pour the blended hot pepper and garlic sauce.
- Add a drizzle of extra virgin olive oil and top with diced tomatoes, and chopped parsley.
- Serve and enjoy with veggies, pitta bread and or olives.

Easy shakshuka recipe

Ingredients

- 2 garlic cloves, peeled, chopped
- 1 large yellow onion, chopped
- Salt and pepper
- ¼ cup chopped fresh mint leaves, 5 grams
- Extra virgin olive oil
- ¼ cup chopped fresh parsley leaves, 5 grams
- 2 green peppers, chopped
- ½ tsp ground cumin
- 6 chopped Vine-ripe tomatoes
- ½ cup tomato sauce
- 1 tsp sweet paprika
- 6 large eggs
- 1 tsp ground coriander
- Pinch red pepper flakes, optional

Directions

- Start by heating 3 teaspoons of olive oil in a saucepan.
- Add onions, garlic, spices, pinch salt, pepper and green peppers.
- Cook while you keep stirring occasionally to soften the veggies for 5 minutes.
- Introduce the tomatoes and tomato sauce together.
- Cover to allow it to simmer for 15 minutes.

- Uncover the content completely to allow it thicken while still cooking.
- Adjust the seasoning according to the taste.
- Make 6 indentation preferably using a wooden spoon in the tomato sauce.
- Break eggs and pour in each of the indentations.
- Reduce the heat, then completely cover the skillet.
- Continue to cook on low heat to set the white eggs
- Uncover and introduce the parsley and mint.
- Serve with warm pita and or add red pepper if desired.
- Enjoy

Italian oven roasted vegetables

The Italian roasted vegetable is a Mediterranean Sea diet that is made out of a variety of veggies. It can be seasoned and using extra virgin olive oil it can be tossed. This recipe is absolutely gluten free.

Ingredients

- Salt and pepper
- 10-12 large peeled garlic cloves
- 8 baby Bella mushrooms with ends trimmed
- Extra virgin olive oil
- 12 oz. baby potatoes, scrubbed
- 12 oz. Campari tomatoes, grape or cherry tomatoes
- 2 zucchini or summer squash, cut into 1-inch pieces
- 1 teaspoon of dried thyme
- ½ teaspoon of dried oregano
- Freshly grated Parmesan cheese for serving, optional
- Crushed red pepper flakes, optional

Directions

- Begin by preheating your oven to 425°.
- Combine the veggies, garlic and the mushrooms in a large bowl and blend.
- Drizzle with the olive oil.

- Add the thyme, pepper, salt, and the dried oregano, then toss to allow it to combine.
- Oil a baking pan to which take the potatoes and spread.
- Roast the potatoes in the heated oven for about 10 minutes or so.
- Remove the potatoes from the heat and introduce the mushrooms along with the vegetables.
- Take it back to the oven for further roasting for 20 minutes.
- Serve immediately with crushed pepper and sprinkle of grated parmesan.
- Enjoy.

Pressure pot borscht

Ingredients

- 2 medium carrots (150 grams)
- 2 celery stalks (200 grams)
- 2 fresh beets (240 grams)
- 3 large potatoes (500 grams)
- 1 onion, medium-large
- 3 garlic cloves
- 4 tablespoons of sour cream
- 2 tablespoons of sunflower oil
- 1.5 cup of water (375 ml)
- 2 tablespoons of white wine vinegar
- 2 bay leaves
- 1 teaspoon of salt
- ¼ teaspoon of black pepper
- 4 cups of vegetable stock (1 liter)
- ¼ cup of tomato puree (50 grams)
- 9 ounces of white cabbage (300 grams)

Directions

- Start by placing oil in to the inner pot of your pressure pot.
- Peel and dice the onion and place into the pot.
- Press the sauté function and set to high.
- Let sauté as you dice the veggies in stages and adding them to the pot.
- Peel the carrots and cut into small pieces.
- When ready, add them to the pot. Stir to mix.

- Trim off the ends of celery then cut each stem in half lengthwise and dice into small pieces.
- Add to the pot and stir to mix.
- Remove the hard part from cabbage and cut.
- Add to the pot and stir to mix.
- Add the beets to the pot and stir again.
- Add tomatoes into the pot, stir and turn off the sauté function.
- Add the remaining ingredients apart from sour cream.
- Lock the lid firmly in its position.
- Turn the steam releasing valve to seal and press cooking.
- Set the timer to 15 minutes and let it cook.
- When ready, wait 10 minutes before releasing pressure manually.
- Serve with a generous dollop of sour cream.
- Enjoy.

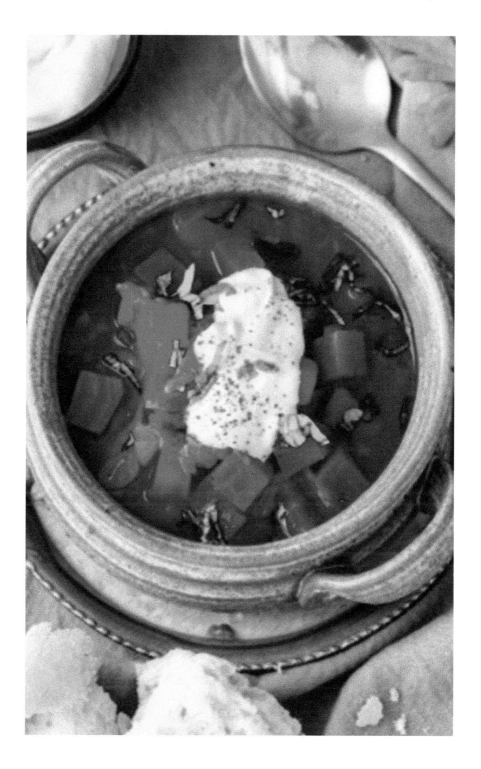

Fresh huevos rancheros

Ingredients

For he Pico de Gallo

- ¼ cup of finely chopped white onion
- ¼ teaspoon of fine-grain sea salt
- 2 medium ripe tomatoes, chopped
- 2 tablespoons of lime juice
- ¼ cup of chopped fresh cilantro

For the refried beans

- Freshly ground black pepper, to taste
- ¼ teaspoon of fine-grain sea salt
- ½ teaspoon of lime juice
- 1 teaspoon of ground cumin
- 2 teaspoons of extra-virgin olive oil
- 1 can of black beans or pinto beans, rinsed and drained
- ¼ cup of water
- ¼ cup of finely chopped white onion

For Everything else

- ½ cup of shredded Monterey Jack cheese
- 1 ½ cups of your favorite red salsa
- Freshly ground black pepper
- 4 teaspoons of extra-virgin olive oil, divided
- 4 corn tortillas
- 4 eggs

Directions

- In a medium bowl, combine the tomatoes together with the onion, cilantro, lime juice, and salt.
- Stir to combine, set the bowl aside for later.
- In a small saucepan over medium heat, warm the olive oil until shimmering but without smoke.
- Add the onions and salt.
- Let cook as you keep stirring occasionally, until the onions have softened in 6 minutes.
- Then, add the cumin to the content let cook for 30 seconds as you keep stirring constantly, until fragrant.
- Pour in the drained beans and water.
- Stir, cover and let cook for 5 minutes.
- Lower the heat, then remove the lid and mash up the beans about half of the beans.
- Let continue to cook the beans when uncovered, stirring often for 3 minutes to thicken.
- Then, remove the pot from the heat source and stir in the pepper and lime juice.
- Taste and adjust accordingly.
- Cover until you are ready to serve.
- Pour the salsa into a medium saucepan over medium heat.

- Bring the salsa to a simmer, stirring occasionally, and then reduce the heat let keep warm until serving.
- In a small skillet over medium heat, warm each tortilla individually, flipping if needed.
- Spread the black bean mixture over each tortilla and place each tortilla on an individual plate. Set aside.
- In the same skillet over medium heat, pour in 1 teaspoon olive oil and wait until it's shimmering but not with smoke.
- Break an egg and pour it into the skillet without breaking the yolk.
- Fry the egg, lifting and tilting the pan occasionally to redistribute the oil, until the whites are set to the preferred level.
- Place the fried egg on top of a prepared tortilla and repeat with the remaining eggs.
- Spoon about ¼ of the warmed salsa across each dish, avoiding the egg yolk.
- Use a slotted spoon to do the same with the Pico de Gallo, without the tomato juices.
- Sprinkle with freshly ground black pepper and add any additional garnishes you might like.
- Serve and enjoy immediately.

Chunky citrus avocado dip

The chunky citrus avocado borrowed the entire Mediterranean style that intrigues the taste buds leaving one to wanting more. This is highly packed with flavors with a fine finishing. Be sure to note that this dip has variations.

Ingredients

- ½ cup/ 60g chopped red onions
- Generous drizzle Early Harvest Greek extra virgin olive oil
- Juice of 1 lime
- 2 large avocados pitted, peeled and diced
- ½ cup chopped cilantro
- Salt and pepper
- ½ cup/ 7g of chopped fresh mint
- Cayenne
- ¾ tsp Sumac
- 1 ¾ or 49g crumbled feta cheese
- 2 Navel oranges, peeled and diced
- ½ cup/400g walnut hearts, chopped

Directions

- Combine red onions, fresh herbs, avocado, oranges, and walnuts in a large bowl.
- Season with pepper, salt, pinch of cayenne, and sumac.

- Drizzle with early harvest extra virgin olive oil after adding lime juice.
- Toss gently to blend and combine
- Add the feta cheese on the top.
- Serve and enjoy with chips of your choice.

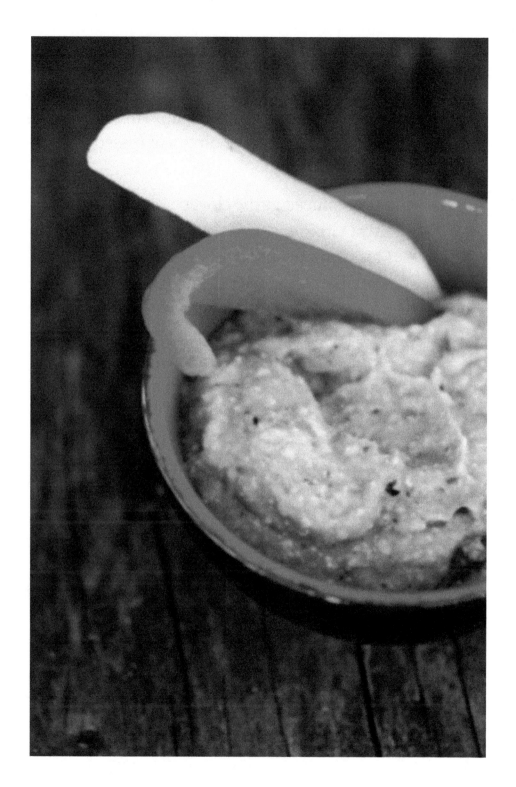

Quick oven roasted tomatoes recipe

There are numerous ways of using the roasted tomatoes as a side dish typically in pasta or soup. This can also be served with bruschetta style or on top of tossed bread.

Ingredients

- 2 or 3 minced garlic cloves
- Extra virgin olive oil
- 1 teaspoon of sumac
- 2 smaller tomatoes cut into halves
- Kosher salt and black pepper
- ½ teaspoon of dry chili pepper flakes
- 2 teaspoons of fresh thyme without stems
- Crumbled feta cheese, optional

Directions

- Start by preheating your oven to 450°.
- Place the tomatoes in a large bowl.
- Add the minced garlic, pepper, salt, thyme and spices.
- Drizzle with extra virgin olive oil, and toss to coat.
- Transfer the tomatoes to a baking sheet that has a rim.
- Spread the tomatoes in one layer with the flesh side facing up.
- Put them in the heated oven for roasting for 30 – 35 minutes.
- Remove off the heat source.

- Garnish with fresh thyme and some sprinkles of feta cheese.
- Serve while warm or at room temperature, depending to what you like.

Roasted cauliflower

This cauliflower recipe is a perfect make especially because of the possibility of combining it with various flavors.

Ingredients

- Handful fresh parsley for garnish optional
- 1 head cauliflower cored and divided into small florets
- ¼ cup/30 g toasted pine nuts or toasted slivered almonds, optional
- 2 teaspoons of ground cumin
- Salt and pepper
- Greek extra virgin olive oil
- 1 to 2 teaspoon of lemon juice or juice of ½ to 1 lemon to your liking
- 1 teaspoon of harissa spice

Directions

- Preheat your oven to 250°.
- Place the cauliflower florets on some large baking sheet.
- To coat the florets, drizzle extra virgin olive oil and toss.
- Add more extra virgin olive oil as needed.
- Combine the harissa and cumin in a small sized dish, then season with the spice mixture and a pinch of black pepper and salt.
- Re-toss to combine and bend

- On the baking sheet evenly spread the cauliflower to form one layer.
- Cover the baking sheet well with a foil and place at the center of preheated oven.
- Roast while covered for 15 minutes.
- Gently remove the foil with care, return the baking sheet to the oven.
- Roast for another 20 – 30 minutes while you keep rotating the baking sheet and cauliflower with a pair of tongs.
- If you intend to serve with tahini, now it is the time to make your tahini.
- Remove the cauliflower from heat and transfer to a serving dish.
- Immediately add lemon juice with some drizzle of tahini, parsley for garnish, and toasted nuts.
- Sprinkle with harissa.
- Serve with tahini as a sauce on the side
- Enjoy.

Easy baked zucchini recipe with thyme and parmesan

With its golden crust, this golden zucchini is fantastic for a crowded pleaser served with some tzatziki sauce. It should be served when still hot to enjoy the best out of it.

Ingredients

- ½ cup grated Parmesan cheese
- 1 teaspoon of dried oregano
- Extra virgin olive oil
- 3 to 4 zucchini trimmed and cut length-wise into quarters
- Pinch kosher salt
- ½ teaspoon of sweet paprika
- ½ teaspoon of black pepper
- 2 teaspoon of fresh thyme leaves no stems

Directions

- Preheat the oven to about 350°
- Mix together the grated Parmesan, thyme and spices until well combined in a small bowl at once.
- Prepare a large baking sheet topped with a wire baking rack.
- Lightly brush the baking rack with extra virgin olive oil.
- Properly arrange the zucchini sticks with the skin side down right on the baking rack.

- Brush every zucchini sticks with extra virgin olive oil
- Sprinkle the Parmesan-thyme topping on each zucchini stick
- Place in the preheated oven for 15 – 20 minutes.
- Broil for 2 to 3 minutes while supervising closely.
- Use tzatziki as an appetizer with a hummus for dipping.
- Serve and enjoy.

Baba gaboughs recipe

This recipe utilizes the taste power in eggplants flavored with garlic, tahini, lime or lemon juice. It is more delicious when served with homemade pita chips.

Ingredients

- Greek extra virgin olive oil
- 1 ½ tablespoon of tahini paste
- ½ teaspoon of sumac, more for garnish
- 1 tablespoon of lime or lemon juice, more if you like
- 1 large eggplant
- ½ teaspoon of cayenne pepper
- Parsley leaves for garnish
- 1 garlic clove
- Salt and pepper
- Toasted pine nuts for garnish
- 1 tablespoon of plain Greek yogurt (optional)

Directions

- Begin by preheat your oven to 425°F.
- Trim the top of the eggplant.
- Using a knife, cut the eggplants in half then make a few slits in its skin.
- Sprinkle the eggplant flesh then allow it to settle for few minutes and dab dry.
- Place the eggplants cut in to halves in an upside down position placed on a baking sheet oiled with drizzle oil.

- Bake in the preheated oven for 30 – 4- minutes until when the eggplants have totally softened.
- Remove it off the heat sauce and let cool.
- After cooling, scoop the flesh out and transfer to a colander and allow it to drain for up to 3 minutes.
- Transfer eggplant to a bowl of a food processor attached with a blade.
- Add tahini, lime juice, yogurt, pepper, salt, cayenne, and sumac.
- Briefly run the food processor to blend the mixture.
- In a small bowl, transfer and spread the baba ganoush.
- Refrigerate while covered for 1 hour to allow the ganoush thicken a little.
- Top the baba ganoush with a sprinkle of sumac right before serving with olive oil, parsley leaves, and toasted pine nuts.
- Enjoy with warm pita bread.

Chicken sharwarma

This sharwarma recipe does not call for unique and special rotisseries to give it sweet delicious taste. Baking it until tender with eastern spices is a perfect way served with pita pockets and other several Mediterranean salads as well as sauces.

Ingredients

- ¾ tablespoon of turmeric powder
- ¾ tablespoon of garlic powder
- ¾ tablespoon of ground coriander
- ¾ tablespoon of paprika
- Salt
- 1 large lemon juice
- ½ teaspoon of ground cloves
- ½ teaspoon of cayenne pepper
- 1/3 cup of extra virgin olive oil
- 1 large thinly sliced onions
- 8 boneless and skinless chicken thighs
- ¾ tablespoon of ground cumin
- 6 pita pockets
- Baby arugula
- Pickles or Kalamata olives
- Tahini sauce
- 3-ingredient Mediterranean salad

Directions

- In a small bowl, mix majority of the ingredients typically the coriander, turmeric, cumin, garlic power, paprika, and cloves.
- Keep the sharwarma spice for later
- Pat the chicken thighs dry and season with salt on both sides.
- Then thinly slice into small bite-sized pieces.
- Put the chicken in a large bowl to Add the shawarma spices, then toss to coat.
- Introduce the onions, olive oil, and lemon juice.
- Toss everything together again.
- Cover totally for refrigeration for up to 3 hours. If there is time for you to wait, refrigerate overnight.
- Preheat your oven to 425 - 430°.
- Transfer the chicken from the fridge to outside and allow it to heat to room temperature for some minutes.
- Spread the marinated chicken with the onions in one layer on a large lightly-oiled baking sheet pan.
- Start to roast in the heated oven for 30 minutes.
- To obtain a proper brown crispy chicken, you can move the pan closer to heat source and briefly while supervising closely.

- As the chicken is still roasting, keep preparing the pitas pockets, make the tahini sauce, tzatziki sauce and the 3-ingredient Mediterranean salad to set side.
- Serve in the pitas by spreading a little tahini sauce or tzatziki sauce .
- Add the chicken shawarma, Mediterranean salad , arugula, and pickles or olives
- Serve immediately and enjoy

Crispy homemade fish sticks

These fish sticks are prepared to be totally tender on the inside and completely crispy on the outside. The seasoning gives it the flavor that anyone is seeking for in any dish or meal. A salmon or white firm fish is just fantastic to make the best of this recipe.

Ingredients

- Parsley garnish
- Salt
- Zest of 1 lemon juice
- ½ of lemon juice for finishing
- ½ cup of bread crumbs
- 1 cup of parmesan
- Extra virgin olive oil
- 1 teaspoon of pepper
- 1 teaspoon of sweet paprika
- 1 teaspoon of totally dried oregano
- 1 ½ lb. of firm fish fillet skinless
- ½ cup of flour
- 1 egg beaten in 1 tablespoon of water
- Tahini sauce

Directions

- Heat your oven to 450°.
- Pat the fish fillet dry and season with kosher salt on either sides.
- Cut the fish fillet into pieces

- Combine the dried oregano, paprika, and the black pepper in a small bowl.
- Season the cut fish fillets on every side with the spice mixture.
- Ensure to make a dredging station, then in a small shallow dish place the flour.
- In a deeper bowl, place the egg wash next to the flour dish. Get a separate dish for combing grated parmesan, bread crumbs, and lemon zest, and place adjacent to the bowl containing the egg wash.
- Coat the fish by dipping them in the flour, shake of the excess flour.
- Deep the fish in the bowl of egg wash.
- From the egg wash bowl, dip it again in the bread crumbs and parmesan mixture.
- Repeat the process until all the fish sticks are coated.
- On an oiled baking sheet, arrange the coated fish, brush extra virgin olive oil. Place the baking sheet in the middle of the already heated oven and bake for 12 - -15 minutes.
- Finish with lemon zest and fresh lemon juice. Garnish with parsley.
- Choose your favorite sauce to serve with either tahini or tzatziki with salad typically Mediterranean white beans salad.
- Enjoy

Falafel recipe

Ingredients

- 7-8 garlic cloves, peeled
- 1 cup fresh parsley leaves, stems removed
- 1 tablespoon of ground cumin
- 1 tablespoon of ground coriander
- 1 teaspoon of cayenne pepper, optional
- Oil for frying
- 1 tablespoon of ground black pepper
- ¾ cup fresh cilantro leaves, stems removed
- 2 tablespoon of toasted sesame seeds
- ½ teaspoon of baking soda
- 1 small onion, quartered
- 2 cups dried chickpeas
- ½ cup fresh dill, stems removed
- Baby Arugula
- Tomatoes, chopped or diced
- Tahini Sauce
- Salt to taste
- Cucumbers, chopped or diced
- 1 teaspoon of baking powder
- Pita pockets
- Pickles

Directions

- 24 hours prior to cooking, place the baking soda and the dried chickpeas in a bowl of water covering the chickpeas by 2 inches.

- Drain the chickpeas when completely soaked, pat dry.
- Add the chickpeas, herbs, onions, garlic and spices to a food processor fitted with a blade.
- Run the food processor for about 40 seconds at a time until all is well combined to form the falafel mixture.
- Change the falafel mixture to a container, then cover tightly for refrigeration for about 1 hour.
- Add the baking powder and sesame seeds right before frying the mixture and stir using a spoon.
- Make patties out of the falafel mixture ½ inch thick.
- Put oil in a medium sized saucepan and heat with a medium temperature to form soft bubbles.
- Place the falafel patties in the oil fry for 3 – 5 minutes until medium brown on the outside.
- In a plate lined with paper, place the falafel to drain the oil.
- While hot, serve the falafel on small plates with pita bread, tomatoes, cucumber or tahini.

Greek-style black eyed peas

The green style black eyed peas are a wonderful recipe to feed a crowd on a limited budget yet healthy and hearty. Onions and garlic with Greek spices give it a flavorful taste when finished with citrus.

Ingredients

- 2 15 ounces cans of black eyed peas, rinsed and drained
- 1 lime or lemon juice
- 1 chopped green bell pepper
- Kosher salt and black pepper
- 1 large chopped yellow onion
- 1 teaspoon of dry oregano
- 1 cup chopped fresh parsley
- 4 chopped garlic cloves
- ½ teaspoon of paprika
- Extra virgin olive oil
- 1 15 ounces of can diced tomato
- 2 cups water
- 1 dry bay leaf
- 2 - 3 carrots, peeled and chopped
- 1 ½ teaspoon of ground cumin
- ½ teaspoon of red pepper flakes, optional

Directions

- In a large pot, heat extra virgin olive oil over medium temperature until shimmering

- Add onions and garlic to Sauté shortly until fragrant and translucent.
- Add bell peppers and carrots and cook for 5 minutes while tossing frequently.
- Add juicy diced tomatoes. Bay leaf, water, salt, spices, and pepper.
- Increase the temperature and let boil.
- Introduce the black eyed peas and boil for 5 minutes after which reduce the heat.
- Cover half-way and let simmer for 25 – 30 minutes.
- Add little water if the stew is too dry
- Stir in the parsley and lemon juice.
- Change to bowels and drizzle with extra virgin olive oil and serve.
- Enjoy with your best grains or warm Greek pita.

Mediterranean-style Juicy salmon burgers

Tired or do not like dry burgers? Enjoy this juicy salmon burger spiced with lemon juice and served with tomatoes and arugula.

Ingredients

- 1 red onion, sliced
- 1 ½ lb. skinless salmon fillet, cut into chunks
- 1 teaspoon of ground sumac
- Bread of your choice (optional)
- ½ teaspoon of black pepper
- 6 baby arugula
- Kosher Salt
- ½ teaspoon of sweet paprika
- Italian bread crumbs for coating
- ¼ cup extra virgin olive oil
- 1 lemon
- 1 cup chopped fresh parsley
- 2-3 tablespoon minced green onions
- Homemade Tzatziki Sauce
- 2 teaspoon of Dijon mustard
- 1 tomato, sliced into rounds
- 1 teaspoon of ground coriander

Directions

- Put ¼ of the salmon in a bowl of a large food processor together with mustard Dijon then run processor to form a pasty mixture

- Move to a bowl.
- Put the remaining salmon in the food processor, and pulse a few times until coarsely chopped into ¼-inch pieces
- Move to the same bowl.
- Add minced green parsley, onions, coriander, paprika, sumac, and black pepper.
- Season with kosher salt, then blend properly until the mixture is totally combined.
- Cover to refrigerate for 30 hours.
- While the salmon chills, prepare the toppings.
- Make the Greek Tzatziki Sauce.
- Prepare the sliced tomatoes, arugula, and the remaining toppings and buns to serve.
- When all these above three parts are ready, bring the salmon out of the fridge.
- Divide into 4 equal parts and form into 1-inch think patties.
- Put bread crumbs on a plate.
- Put each patty in the bread crumbs plate, then coat on both sides.
- Move the breaded salmon patties on a sheet pan lined with parchment paper.
- Cook salmon patties.
- Heat 3 tablespoons of extra virgin olive oil over medium temperature until shimmering without smoke.

- Bring down the salmon patties gently continue to cook for 2 – 4 minutes while turning over once until when lightly brown on all sides. Regulate the temperature as necessary.
- Arrange cooked salmon burgers onto paper towel to drain any excess oil
- Sprinkle lightly if you desire with Kosher salt.
- Squeeze of fresh lemon juice on top.
- Assemble in prepared buns.
- Spread the buns with a bit of tzatziki sauce.
- Add the salmon, then layer on the arugula, onion slices, and tomato
- Serve and enjoy

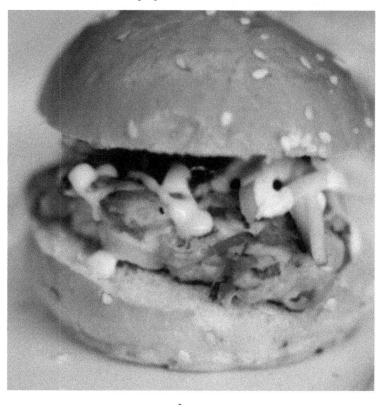

Greek-style eggplant recipe

Greek-style eggplant recipe is a total meatless velvet prepared with chickpeas and tomatoes. It can serve as dinner or just side dish with the delicious satisfaction that everyone is seeking for.

Ingredients

- 1.5 lb. eggplant, cut into cubes
- 1 teaspoon of organic ground coriander
- Fresh herbs such as parsley and mint for garnish
- 1 28 ounces can of chopped tomato
- 2 15 ounces cans chickpeas, reserve the canning liquid
- 6 large garlic cloves, minced
- ½ teaspoon of black pepper
- 2 dry bay leaves
- Kosher salt
- 1 large yellow onion, chopped
- 1 green bell pepper, stem and innards removed and diced
- ½ teaspoon of organic ground turmeric
- Extra Virgin Olive Oil
- 1 carrot, chopped
- 1 to 1 ½ tsp sweet paprika OR smoked paprika
- ¾ teaspoon of ground cinnamon
- 1 teaspoon of dry oregano

Directions

- Preheat the oven to 400°.
- Put cut eggplant cubes in a colander over a large bowl to sprinkle with salt.
- Keep aside for 20 minutes to give room for the eggplant to "sweat out" any bitterness.
- Rinse with water, then pat dry.
- Heat ¼ cup of extra virgin olive oil over medium to shimmer.
- Add peppers, onions, and chopped carrot allow to cook for 2 – 3 minutes while constantly stirring.
- Add garlic, spices, bay leaf, and a dash of salt.
- Let cook for another minute keeping stirring until fragrant.
- Add the chickpeas, eggplant, chopped tomato, reserved chickpea liquid and stir to blend.
- Cook at a rolling point for 10 minutes.
- Remove from stove top, cover and move to oven.
- Continue to cook in oven for 45 minutes until eggplant is totally cooked.
- Remove from oven when ready
- Add a drizzle of extra virgin olive oil, parsley or mint.
- Serve hot with side Greek yogurt, pita bread or tzatziki sauce.

Easy Moroccan vegetable tagine

This is a simple vegan packed vegetable stew with several Moroccan flavors. It is entirely gluten free; thus healthy.

Ingredients

- 1 teaspoon of ground coriander
- 1-quart low-sodium vegetable broth
- 2 large carrots, peeled and chopped
- 2 large russet potatoes, peeled and cubed
- ½ cup heaping chopped dried apricot
- 1 large sweet potato, peeled and cubed
- Salt
- ¼ cup extra virgin olive oil, more for later
- 2 medium yellow onions, peeled and chopped
- Handful fresh parsley leaves
- 1 tablespoon Harissa spice blend
- 8 – 10 garlic cloves, peeled and chopped
- 1 teaspoon of ground cinnamon
- 1 lemon, juice of
- 2 cups canned whole peeled tomatoes
- ½ teaspoon of ground turmeric
- 2 cups cooked chickpeas

Directions

- In a heavy large pot, heat olive oil over medium heat until shimmering.
- Add onions and increase the temperature to medium-high.

- Sauté for 5 minutes while tossing frequently.
- Add garlic and all chopped veggies to the solution, then Season with salt and spices, then toss again to combine.
- Cook for about 5 – 7 minutes on medium-high temperature stirring regularly.
- Add apricot, tomatoes, and broth. Season with a small dash of salt.
- Keep the heat on medium allow to cook for 10 minutes.
- Lower the heat, cover properly and let simmer for 20 – 25 minutes until veggies are tender.
- Stir in chickpeas cook for 5 minutes on low heat.
- Introduce the lemon juice and fresh parsley while stirring.
- Taste and adjust seasoning.
- Transfer to serving bowls and top each with a generous drizzle of extra virgin olive oil.
- Serve hot with rice, bread or couscous.

Simple Mediterranean olive pasta

The Mediterranean olive pasta is fully loaded with Mediterranean Sea diet flavors. It derives its sweet taste from this flavors.

Ingredients

- Zest of 1 lemon
- 6 ounces of marinated artichoke hearts, drained
- 1 lb. thin spaghetti
- ¼ cup pitted olives, halved
- ¼ cup crumbled feta cheese, more if you like
- 12 ounces of grape tomatoes, halved
- 1 cup chopped fresh parsley
- 1 teaspoon black pepper
- ½ cup early harvest Greek extra virgin olive oil
- Salt
- 10-15 fresh basil leaves, torn
- 4 garlic cloves, crushed
- 3 scallions of green onions, top trimmed, all whites and greens chopped
- Crushed red pepper flakes (optional)

Directions

- Cook thin spaghetti pasta to al dente according to package instruction.
- Heat the extra virgin olive oil in a large cast iron skillet over medium heat When pasta is almost cooked.

- Reduce the heat immediately add garlic and a pinch of salt.
- Cook briefly for 10 seconds keep stirring regularly.
- Stir in the parsley, chopped scallions, and tomatoes.
- Over low heat, Cook until just warmed through for 30 seconds.
- Remove from heat, when ready and drain off extra cooking water.
- Return to the cooking pot.
- Add the warmed olive oil sauce in toss to coat.
- Toss again to coat after adding black pepper.
- Add all the remaining ingredients and toss.
- Immediately serve in pasta bowls.
- Top each with more basil leaves and feta
- Enjoy!

Mediterranean roasted vegetable barley

This utilizes the sweetness magic in fresh herbs, citrus and extra virgin olive oil to trick one's taste buds.

Ingredients

- Water
- 2 whole zucchini squash and diced
- Early Harvest Greek extra virgin olive oil
- 1 garlic clove, minced
- 1 163 g dry pearl barley, washed
- 2 scallions of green onions, trimmed and chopped
- 1 medium red onion and diced
- 1 yellow bell pepper, cored and diced
- 1 red bell pepper, cored and diced
- salt and pepper
- 2 teaspoon of harissa spice , divided
- ¾ teaspoon of smoked paprika , divided
- 2 tablespoon of fresh squeezed lemon juice
- 56 g chopped fresh parsley
- Toasted pine nuts (optional)
- Feta cheese

Instruction

- Preheat your oven to 425°.
- In a saucepan, put pearl barley and 2 ½ cups water.
- Boil, then reduce the heat to low.
- Cover and cook for 40 – 45 minutes.

- As the barley cooks, add all diced vegetables on a large baking sheet.
- Season with salt, pepper, 1 ½ teaspoon of harissa spice, and ½ teaspoon of smoked paprika.
- Drizzle with extra virgin olive oil and toss to coat.
- Spread evenly in one layer on the baking sheet.
- Roast in the heated oven for 25 minutes.
- Drain the excess water when barley is ready.
- Season again with salt, pepper, ½ teaspoon of harissa spice and ¼ teaspoon of smoked paprika toss again to make sure it combines.
- Move the barley to a large mixing bowl.
- Add roasted veggies.
- Add chopped garlic, scallions, and fresh parsley.
- Dress with lemon juice
- Drizzle with Early Harvest extra virgin olive oil and Toss.
- If desired, top with toasted pine nuts and crumbled feta.
- Serve warm, cold or at room temperature.
- Enjoy

Couscous recipe

In only 15 minutes, you can make couscous recipe with handful ingredients. Couscous serves as the best side next to your favorite protein or exciting bed to a tasty stew as desired.

Ingredients

- 1 cup dry instant couscous
- 1 cup low-sodium broth or water
- Extra virgin olive oil
- Kosher Salt
- Fresh herbs to your liking, optional
- Pinch of cumin optional
- 2 green onions, chopped, optional
- 1 – 2 garlic clove, minced, Sautéed in an extra virgin olive oil, optional

Directions

- Add broth or water in a saucepan.
- Add a drizzle of extra virgin olive oil together with a pinch of kosher salt.
- Bring to a boil.
- Toast the couscous.
- Heat 1 – 2 tablespoon of extra virgin olive oil.
- Add the couscous and toss around with a wooden spoon for it to turn golden brown to add desired flavor. Optional
- Stir in the couscous quickly and turn the heat off soon enough.

- Cover and let settle for 10 minutes for the couscous to absorbed all the water.
- Uncover and fluff with a fork.
- Serve couscous plain.
- To flavor it up mix in spices and herbs.
- If desired, add in a pinch of cumin, chopped green onions, Sautéed garlic, and fresh herbs
- Enjoy.

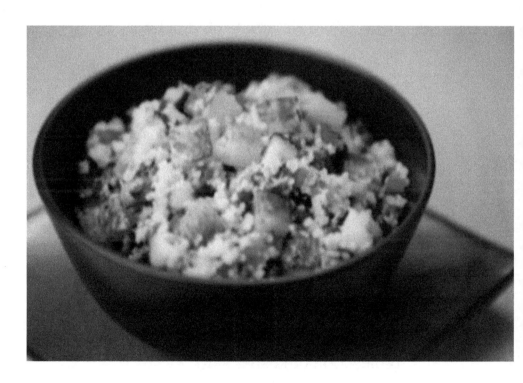

Mediterranean-style tuna pasta

20 minutes is just sufficient to make this darn delicious tuna pasta with highly bold flavors. The ingredients are quite simple ingredients typically parsley, lemon zest parmesan and others listed below.

Ingredients

- ½ lemon juice
- 1 ½ cups frozen peas
- 1 red bell pepper, cored and cut into thin strips
- Black pepper
- 6 garlic cloves, minced
- 6 – 8 pitted Kalamata olives sliced
- Extra virgin olive oil
- Zest of 1 lemon
- ¾ lb. spaghetti
- Handful chopped fresh parsley
- 1 tsp dried oregano
- 2 – 5 ounces of cans solid albacore tuna, drained
- Grated Parmesan cheese
- Kosher salt
- 1 sliced jalapeno pepper (optional)

Directions

- Boil 3 quarts of water to a rolling boil with 1 tablespoon of kosher salt.
- Cook the pasta in the boiling water as per the package Directions

- Add the frozen peas to the cooked pasta continue to cook for the remaining time about 2 – 4 minutes.
- Take ¾ cup of the cooking water and set it aside after the pasta is ready.
- Drain the water in the pasta and peas in a colander.
- In a deep large cooking pan, heat 2 tablespoons of extra virgin olive oil over medium temperature to shimmering without smoke.
- Introduce the red bell peppers
- Cook for 3 – 4 minutes while tossing frequently.
- Add the garlic cook and toss again frequently for 30 seconds until fragrant.
- It is the right time to add the cooked pasta and peas to the pan and toss to combine.
- Add the lemon zest, jalapeno, tuna, parsley, lemon juice, oregano, black pepper, Kalamata olives, and heavy sprinkle of Parmesan cheese.
- Drizzle a small extra virgin olive oil and pasta cooking water as necessary.
- Toss everything.
- Taste and adjust seasoning accordingly
- Serve the pasta and enjoy.

Greek lemon rice

Onions, lemon juice, garlic, and fresh herbs give this meal a wonderful flavor. These flavors have made Greek lemon rice a favorite dinner meal for many individuals and families.

Ingredients

- Early Harvest Greek extra virgin olive oil
- Pinch salt
- 1 garlic clove, minced
- 1 teaspoon of dry dill weed
- 1 zest of lemon
- 2 lemons
- Large handful chopped fresh parsley
- 2 cups of raw long grain rice
- ½ cup orzo pasta
- 1 medium yellow onion, chopped
- 2 cups low sodium broth

Directions

- Thoroughly wash the rice, then soak it for approximately 15 – 20 minutes in cold water sufficient enough to fully immerse the rice at least by 1 inch.
- Drain out all the water
- In a large sauce pan with a lid, heat 3 tablespoons of extra virgin olive oil to shimmer without smoke.
- Add onions and cook for 3 – 4 minutes until when it becomes translucent.

- Then add the garlic together with the orzo pasta.
- Toss shortly to give the orzo some color then stir in the rice continue to toss to coat.
- Introduce the broth and lemon juice let the liquid to boil at a rolling boil point.
- Lower the heat, keep rice covered and cook for about 20 minutes.
- Remove rice from heat.
- Let it simmer for about 10 minutes for better outcome and taste.
- Uncover and stir in dill weed, parsley, and lemon zest.
- Garnish with lemon on top.
- Enjoy.

Lebanese rice with vermicelli

Ingredients

- ½ cup toasted pine nuts, to finish, though optional
- Water
- 2 cups of long grain
- 1 cup broken vermicelli pasta
- Salt
- 2 ½ tablespoon of olive oil

Directions

- Ultimately, start by rinsing the rice properly.
- Put the rinsed rice in a medium bowl and cover with water let soak for 15 – 20 minutes.
- Make sure you are able to easily break the grain of rice with your thumbs, drain all the water.
- Heat the olive oil on medium temperature in a medium non-stick cooking pot.
- Add the vermicelli and continuously stir to equally toast it.
- Make sure the vermicelli should transform to a golden brown color with intensive supervision to prevent burning.
- Add the rice and continue to stir so that the rice will be well-coated with the olive oil.
- Season with salt.
- Add 3 ½ cups of water and bring it to a boil until the water reduces in size.

- Reduce the heat significantly low and keep the rice covered.
- Continue to cook for 15 – 20 minutes on that low heat.
- When the rice is completely cooked switch off the heat
- Simmer the rice for 10 – 15 minutes in its pot.
- Uncover and fluff with a fork
- Serve and top with toasted pine nuts.
- Enjoy.

Greek style baked cod with lemon and garlic

In only 15 minutes you would have finished to bake this Greek style cod with lemon and garlic with handful of spices and much garlic to give it an attractive aroma and taste.

Ingredients

- ½ teaspoon of black pepper
- ¾ teaspoon of sweet Spanish paprika
- 1.5 lb. Cod fillet pieces about 4 or 6 pieces
- 5 tablespoons of fresh lemon juice
- 5 peeled and minced garlic cloves
- 1 teaspoon of ground coriander
- ¾ teaspoon of ground cumin
- 2 tablespoons of melted butter
- ¼ cup chopped fresh parsley leaves
- 5 tablespoons of Private Reserve extra virgin olive oil
- ⅓ cup all-purpose flour
- ¾ teaspoon of salt

Directions

- Preheat oven to 400°F.
- After, mix the lemon juice with olive oil, and melted butter in a shallow bowl.
- Keep aside, safely.

- In a separate second shallow bowl, mix all-purpose flour, salt, spices, and pepper, then also set a side just next to the lemon juice mixture.
- Pat fish the fillet dry.
- To coat, dip fish in the lemon juice mixture, and also dip in the flour mixture.
- Endeavor to shake off any excess flour.
- Keep the remaining lemon juice mixture for later.
- In a cast iron skillet, heat 2 teaspoon of olive oil over medium-high temperature to until shimmering without smoke.
- Add fish and sear on both side to give color. Cook for few minutes on every side.
- Take off the heat.
- Add minced garlic to the remaining lemon juice mixture and blend.
- Then drizzle all over the fish fillets.
- Bake in the heated oven for 10 minutes or until it begins to flake easily when tapped with a fork.
- Take off the heat and sprinkle with chopped parsley.
- Serve immediately preferable with Lebanese rice, traditional Greek salad or any other salad of your choice.
- Enjoy.

One pan Mediterranean baked halibut with vegetables recipe

This exact halibut is made simply with green beans and cherry tomatoes in only 25 minutes. Citrus, fresh garlic and other spices give it a flavorful delicious taste to shake one's taste buds.

Ingredients

- ½ - ¾ teaspoon of ground coriander
- Zest of 2 lemons
- 1 teaspoon of seasoned salt, more for later
- 1 lb. cherry tomatoes
- 1 ½ lb. halibut fillet, sliced into about 1 ½-inch pieces
- 1 ½ tablespoon of freshly minced garlic
- ½ teaspoon of ground black pepper
- 1 cup Private Reserve Greek extra virgin olive oil
- 1 teaspoon of dried oregano
- 1 lb. fresh green beans
- 2 teaspoon of dill weed
- Juice of 2 lemons
- 1 large yellow onion sliced into half moons

Directions

- Preheat your oven to 425°F.
- Begin by whisking the sauce ingredients together, in a large mixing bowl.

- Add the green tomatoes, beans, and onions toss to coat with the whisked sauce
- Using a large slotted spoon, move the vegetables to a large baking sheet
- Keep the vegetables to one side of the baking sheet. Spread out in only one layer.
- You can proceed to add the halibut fillet strips to the remaining sauce then toss to enabling coating.
- Move the halibut fillet to the baking sheet right next to the vegetables.
- Pour any remaining sauce on top.
- Lightly sprinkle the halibut and vegetables with seasoned salt.
- Start to bake in the already heated oven for 15 minutes.
- Move the baking sheet to the top oven rack
- Broil for more 3 minutes with close supervision to prevent burning until when the cherry tomatoes pop right under the broiler.
- Remove the baked halibut and vegetables from the oven when ready
- Serve and enjoy.

Moroccan fish recipe

An equivalent of braised cod recipe, the Moroccan fish recipe is a game changer in regards to sweetness and deliciousness of this recipe. Made in thick tomato sauce, chickpea and pepper with several other healthy Moroccan Mediterranean flavors, you do not want to miss out on this recipe; try out for yourself.

Ingredients

- 1 ½ lb. cod fillet pieces
- 1 ½ cup water
- Extra Virgin Olive Oil
- ½ teaspoon of cumin
- 2 tablespoon of tomato paste
- ½ lemon juice
- ½ lemon, sliced into thin rounds
- 2 medium tomatoes, diced
- 1 red pepper, cored, sliced
- ¾ teaspoon of paprika
- 1 15-oz. can chickpeas, drained and rinsed
- Kosher salt and black pepper
- Large handful fresh cilantro
- 8 garlic cloves, divided minced and sliced 4 for each
- 1 ½ teaspoon of Ras El Hanout , should be divided

Directions

- In a large pan with cover, start by heating 2 tablespoons of extra virgin olive oil over medium temperature until shimmering without smoke.
- Add minced garlic let cook shortly of course while tossing frequently until fragrant.
- Add diced tomato, tomato paste, and bell peppers continue to cook for 3 – 4 minutes in a medium temperature and again keep tossing frequently.
- Add water, cilantro, chickpeas, and sliced garlic let season with kosher salt and pepper.
- Stir in ½ teaspoon of Ras El Hanout spice mixture.
- Increase the heat and boil.
- Bring down the heat and cover part-way an let simmer for 20 minutes. It is absolutely okay to add water if necessary.
- Whereas, combine the remaining cumin with Ras El Hanout , paprika in a small bowl.
- Season the fish with kosher salt and pepper and the spice mixture on either sides.
- Add a drizzle of the extra virgin olive oil.
- Check to see that all the fish is properly coated with the spices and the olive oil.

- Add the season fish to the pan, when ready, then nestle the fish pieces into the saucy chickpea and tomato mixture.
- Add lemon juice and lemon slices.
- Cook content for more 10 − 15 minutes on a low temperature until content is completely cooked.
- Garnish with fresh cilantro.
- Serve as soon as possible with crusty bread or rice.

Baked chicken recipe

No doubt chicken is one of the world's favorite dishes that is deliciously enjoyed by millions to billions of people. The baked chicken uses spicy garlic and fresh basil as well as parsley to keep you hanging on the dish forever.

Ingredients

- 1 medium red onion, halved and thinly sliced
- 44.4 ml Extra virgin olive oil
- 5 – 6 Campari tomatoes halved
- Fresh basil leaves for garnish
- Juice of ½ lemon
- Salt and pepper
- 3.6 g dry oregano
- 1 teaspoon of fresh thyme
- 907.185g of boneless skinless chicken breast
- 2.1g Sweet paprika
- 4 garlic cloves, minced
- Handful chopped fresh parsley for garnish

Directions

- Begin by preheating your oven to 425°.
- Firstly, pat the chicken dry.
- Put the chicken breast in a large zip-top then zip it after releasing air that might be in bag.
- Put it on a poultry chopping board, pound with meat mallet until the chicken flattens.

- Remove out of the zip-top bag, repeat the process with all the remaining chicken breast pieces.
- Season chicken with salt and pepper on every side, then put in a large mixing bowl.
- Add spices, extra virgin olive oil, minced garlic, and lemon juice.
- Combine to ensure the chicken is equally coated with the spices and garlic.
- Oil a large baking dish very lightly, then spread onion slices on the bottom.
- Organize seasoned chicken on top after which add the tomatoes to it.
- Tightly cover the baking dish with a foil let bake for 10 minutes.
- Then uncover, continue to bake for more 8 – 10 minutes. Nevertheless, this step may take more that the specified time according to the thickness of your chicken breast.
- Take off the source of heat.
- Keep covered with a pan for more 5 – 10 minutes before you serve
- Uncover and garnish with fresh parsley and basil.
- Serve and enjoy

Mediterranean shrimp recipe

The shrimp is perfectly coated in Mediterranean spices with skillet cooked in a tasty white wine olive oil sauce that contains shallots, tomatoes and peppers. This should take less than 25 minutes and its ready for you bite.

Ingredients

- 1 ¼ lb. large shrimp peeled and deveined
- 1 tablespoon of butter
- 3 tablespoons of Private Reserve extra virgin olive oil
- 1 Lebanese Rice recipe
- ½ teaspoon of ground coriander
- 2 tablespoons of dry white wine
- ½ teaspoon of each salt and pepper
- 4 garlic cloves, chopped
- ½ green bell pepper
- 2 teaspoons of smoked Spanish paprika
- ⅓ cup chopped parsley leaves
- 1 tablespoon of all-purpose flour
- ¼ teaspoon of cayenne
- 1 cup canned diced tomato
- ⅓ cup chicken or vegetable broth
- ¼ teaspoon of sugar
- 3 shallots thinly sliced
- ½ yellow bell pepper sliced
- 2 tablespoons of fresh lemon juice

Directions

- Start by preparing the Lebanese rice as per the package Directions.
- Keep covered and undisturbed until ready to serve.
- Pat shrimp dry then put it in a large bowl.
- Add flour, salt, smoked paprika, pepper, cayenne, coriander, and sugar.
- Toss until shrimp is fully coated on all sides.
- In a large heavy frying pan, heat to melt the butter together with the olive oil over medium temperature.
- Introduce the shallots and garlic to the content let cook for 2 – 3 minutes as you stir till fragrant.
- Add bell peppers continue to cook for more 4 minutes while tossing infrequently.
- Place the shrimp in the content and cook for 1 – 2 minutes.
- Add the diced broth, tomatoes, white wine and lemon juice.
- Let cook for 5 minutes till when the shrimp turns bright orange.
- Stir in chopped fresh parsley.
- Serve soon enough with the cooked rice you started with.
- Enjoy.

Baked lemon garlic salmon recipe

Ingredients

- Zest of 1 large lemon
- Extra virgin olive oil
- Kosher salt
- Parsley for garnish
- 5 garlic cloves, chopped
- 2 teaspoon of dry oregano
- ½ lemon, sliced into rounds
- 1 teaspoon of sweet paprika
- 2 lb. salmon fillet
- 3 tablespoon of extra virgin olive oil
- Juice of 2 lemons
- ½ teaspoon of black pepper

Directions

- Begin by heating your oven to 375 °.
- Secondly, make the lemon-garlic sauce.
- In a small bowl, mix together the lemon zest, lemon juice, oregano, extra virgin olive oil, garlic, paprika and black pepper.
- Whisk the sauce to perfection.
- Organize your sheet pan lined with a large piece of foil that can fold over to cover the salmon.
- Brush top of the foil with extra virgin olive oil.
- Pat salmon dry, then season properly on all sides with kosher salt.
- Put it on the foiled sheet pan.

- Top with the already made lemon garlic sauce.
- Fold foil over the salmon covering the whole salmon.
- Let bake for 15 – 20 minutes until salmon is about to be cooked through at the thickest part. Nonetheless, the 15 – 20 minutes is directly dependent on the thickness of the salmon.
- Be vigilant to ensure that it is not over cooked.
- Gently, remove from oven, open foil to uncover the top of the salmon.
- Briefly put salmon under the broiler for 3 minutes.
- Make sure the garlic does not burn due to over broiling.
- Serve and enjoy.

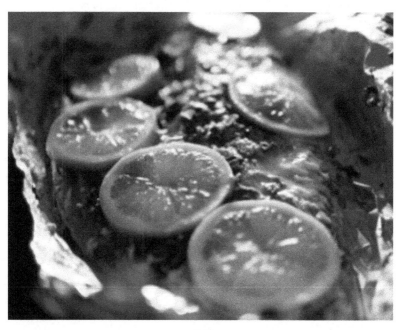

Sheet pan chicken and vegetables

This chicken is a perfect combination with vegetables and no fuss but tossed with oregano, citrus, and of course garlic that masterminds the flavor and unique taste. This vegetable chicken is a beautifully sweet and healthy option for Mediterranean diet lovers.

Ingredients

- Extra virgin olive oil
- 1 large red pepper, cored and cut to chunks
- 1 teaspoon of Paprika
- 1 lemon, zested and juiced
- 2 teaspoon of dry oregano
- 1 teaspoon of white vinegar
- 1 red onion, cut into chunks
- 9 baby broccoli, trimmed and cut into equal pieces
- 1 ½ lb. boneless chicken breast
- 1 teaspoon of coriander
- 5 garlic cloves, minced
- Kosher salt and black pepper
- 2 medium zucchini halved length-wise, sliced into crescent shape of a moon
- Fresh parsley for garnish, optional

Directions

- Heat your oven to about 400°.
- Put all the cut vegetables in a large mixing bowl.

- Then add chicken pieces together with the minced garlic.
- Season with kosher salt and black pepper.
- Add spices.
- Add lemon juice, lemon zest, vinegar, drizzle generously with extra virgin olive oil.
- Toss properly to ensure perfect combining. Furthermore, endeavor to ensure that the vegetables and chicken pieces are equally coated.
- Move content to a large sheet pan and spread well in only one layer.
- Begin baking in the ready heated oven for 20 minutes or until the chicken is totally cooked through.
- You can garnish with fresh parsley before you continue to serve.
- Enjoy.

Sicilian style fish stew recipe

This Mediterranean diet dish is packed with Italian flavors to heighten its delicacy. It is best in white wine-tomato broth, capers and garlic among other ingredients.

Ingredients

- Salt
- Pepper
- ¾ cup of dry white wine
- 4 large garlic cloves, minced
- ½ teaspoon dried thyme
- 2 lb. skinless sea bass fillet cut into large cubes
- Crusty Italian bread for serving
- ¼ cup of golden raisins
- Pinch red pepper flakes
- 1 large yellow onion, chopped
- 2 tablespoon of rinsed capers
- ½ cup chopped fresh parsley leaves
- 2 celery ribs, chopped
- 3 cups of low-sodium vegetable broth
- Extra virgin olive oil
- 1 28-oz. can of whole peeled plum tomatoes, juice separated and reserved
- 3 tablespoons of toasted pine nuts, optional

Directions

- Start by heating 1 tablespoon of olive oil in 5-quart oven over medium temperature.

- Add celery, onions, and a small salt and pepper.
- Cook while regularly stirring until softened in for 4 minutes.
- Add thyme, red pepper flakes and garlic continue to cook shortly until fragrant enough only in 30.
- Stir in the white wine and reserved tomato juice from a can.
- Simmer briefly then continue cooking until the liquid reduces significantly by ½.
- Add the vegetable broth, tomatoes, raisins, and capers.
- Cook for more 15 – 20 minutes on a medium temperature until flavors are fully combined.
- Pat the fish dry, then proceed to season lightly with the salt and pepper.
- Carefully fix pieces of fish into the already cooking liquid then stir gently to nicely cover the fish pieces in the cooking liquid.
- Simmer for some time, continue to cook for more 5 minutes.
- Remove content from source of heat and cover.
- Let settle off heat for more 4 – 5 minutes to ensure swift cooking of all the pieces of fish.

- Make sure the fish is flaky enough when gently pulled apart from the sauce with a knife or fork.
- Lastly, you can stir in the chopped parsley.
- Pour the hot fish stew into serving bowls immediately to top with toasted pine nuts if desired.
- Serve with crusty bread
- Enjoy.

Greek chicken souvlaki with tzatziki

Believe me not, this recipe will remind you of the last time you had it for dinner in streets of Athens. You most likely would want to make your own because you are now far away from their yet the taste of this amazing recipe keeps calling your name. below are the ingredients and complete step-by-step Directions.

Ingredients

- 2 bay leaves
- Greek pita bread
- Sliced tomato
- 1 teaspoon of each Kosher salt and black pepper
- Tzatziki Sauce
- ¼ cup dry white wine
- Juice of 1 lemon
- 2 ½ lb.. of organic boneless skinless chicken breast, no fats and cut into 1 ½ inch pieces
- 2 tablespoons of dried oregano
- 10 garlic cloves, peeled
- sliced cucumber
- 1 teaspoon of dried rosemary
- ¼ cup of Greek extra virgin olive oil
- sliced onions
- Kalamata olives
- 1 teaspoon of sweet paprika

Directions

- Begin by preparing the marinade.
- In a small food processor bowl, add oregano, pepper, garlic, paprika, rosemary, salt, white wine, olive oil, and lemon juice, then pulse thoroughly to combine.
- Add bay leaves to chicken put in a separate large bowl.
- Top it with marinade toss thoroughly to ensure that it is fully combined.
- Ensure chicken is properly and evenly coated.
- Cover tightly and refrigerate for 2 hours
- Get 10 – 12 wooden skewers, then soak properly in water for 30 – 45 minutes.
- Proceed to prepare the tzatziki sauce including all other fixings.
- Thread marinated chicken pieces through the prepared skewers when the tzatziki sauce is ready.
- Organize the outdoor grill
- Brush with a small oil and heat over medium temperature.
- Put the chicken skewers on grill until well browned, keeping regulating inside temperature around 155° on the monitoring thermometer for 5 minutes.
- Keeping brushing with marinade, discard any leftovers.

- Move the chicken to serving area let cool for 3 minutes.
- Warm the pitas through.
- Arrange chicken souvlaki pitas after spreading with tzatziki sauce on the pita, add chicken pieces and lastly add the vegetables and olives.
- Enjoy.

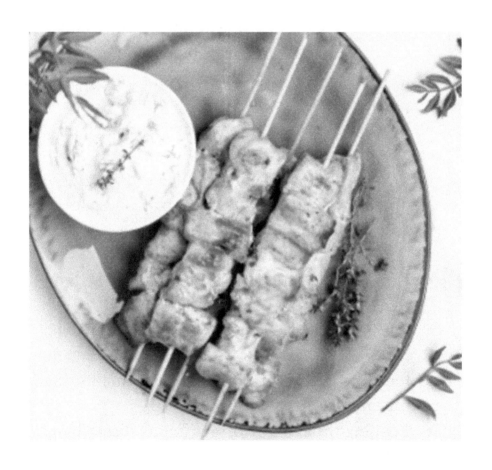

Grilled swordfish with a Mediterranean twist

The swordfish recipe highly relies on the delicious marinade of the Mediterranean pumped with fresh garlic cloves, cumin among others flavorful ingredients. Try to make this at home with the following ingredients and step-by-step directions below.

Ingredients

- 4 swordfish steaks
- ¾ teaspoon of cumin
- ½ tsp freshly ground black pepper
- ⅓ cup extra virgin olive oil
- 6 to 12 garlic cloves, peeled
- ½ to 1 tsp sweet Spanish paprika
- 1 teaspoon of coriander
- ¾ teaspoon of salt
- 2 tablespoon of fresh lemon juice
- Crushed red pepper, optional

Directions

- Begin by blending the olive oil, garlic, spices, lemon juice, salt and pepper in a food processor for 3 minutes.
- Pat the swordfish steaks dry
- Place the dry swordfish steaks in a pan to generously apply the marinade on every side

after which keep aside for 15 minutes as the grill heats up

- Oil the grates and preheat a gas grill with high temperature.
- When properly heat, grill the fish steaks on high temperature for 5 – 6 minutes on one side and so the other side until the fish can easily flake when tapped with a fork.
- Use a splash of lemon juice to finish and sprinkle with crushed red pepper flakes as desired.
- Serve and enjoy.

Greek shrimp recipe with tomato and feta

The flavors in this recipe are fully packed. It includes fresh herbs, tomato sauce, feta as well as olive. This dish is served with crusty bread or even favorite grains.

Ingredients

- 1 ½ teaspoon of dry dill weed, divided
- Pinch red pepper flakes
- 2 56g crumbled Greek feta cheese
- 6 garlic cloves, minced, divided
- 1 ½ teaspoon of dry oregano, divided
- Chopped fresh mint leaves
- Greek extra virgin olive oil
- Juice of ½ lemon
- Black pepper
- 6 pitted Kalamata olives, optional
- 1 large red onion, chopped
- 1 ½ lb. large shrimp fully thawed, peeled and deveined
- Kosher salt
- 1 737.088g canned diced tomato, drain only some of the liquid
- Chopped fresh parsley leaves

Directions

- Pat shrimp dry, put in a large bowl.
- Season with kosher pepper, salt, ½ teaspoon of dry oregano, pinch red pepper flakes, ½

teaspoon of dry dill weed, and ½ teaspoon of minced garlic.

- Drizzle with the extra virgin olive oil
- Toss thoroughly to fully combine keep aside.
- In a large skillet, heat 2 teaspoon of extra virgin olive oil on medium heat until shimmering without smoke.
- Add chopped onion together with all the remaining minced garlic then cook shortly while stirring frequently until fragrant.
- Add tomatoes together with the lemon juice
- Season with a pinch of pepper, salt, dill, and the remaining dry oregano.
- Boil
- Reduce the heat to medium to allow simmering for 15 minutes.
- Introduce the marinated shrimp.
- Continue to cook for 5 – 7 minutes
- Now it is time to stir in fresh mint and parsley leaves.
- Sprinkle the feta and black olives to finish.
- If desired, add a splash of lemon juice according to your taste preference.
- Serve over plain orzo or your favorite crusty bread.
- Enjoy.

Mediterranean sautéed shrimp and zucchini

Ingredients

- 1 teaspoon of ground coriander
- 1 lb. large shrimp
- ½ teaspoon of sweet paprika
- Kosher salt
- 1 ½ cups cherry tomatoes, halved
- Handful fresh basil leaves, torn or sliced into ribbons
- ½ medium red onion, thinly sliced
- 5 garlic cloves, minced and divided
- Extra virgin olive oil
- 2 zucchini halved and sliced into ½ moons
- 1 teaspoon of ground cumin
- 1 ½ tablespoon of dry oregano
- Pepper
- 1 cup cooked chickpeas drained
- 1 bell pepper, cored and sliced into sticks
- 1 large lemon juice

Directions

- Combine cumin, coriander, oregano, and paprika in a small bowl.
- Pat shrimp dry and season with 1 ½ tsp of the spice mixture and kosher salt.

- Set aside in a refrigerator mainly if you will use at a later time. Ensure to keep some spice mixture for the veggies.
- Heat 2 tablespoon of extra virgin olive oil over medium temperature in a large cast iron skillet.
- Add½ the amount of garlic together with the onions let cook for 3 – 4 minutes keep tossing regularly until fragrant.
- Add the bell peppers, zucchini, and chickpeas together for seasoning with pepper and salt together with the remaining spice mixture.
- Toss to combine and blend.
- Increase the heat if deemed necessary continue to cook the veggies until tender of course keep tossing regularly for 5 – 7 minutes.
- Move all the vegetable to large plate for the moment.
- Take back the skillet to the heat, add small extra virgin olive oil.
- Add the seasoned shrimp and remaining garlic.
- Cook over medium temperature while stirring occasionally in 4 – 5 minutes till shrimp is totally pink
- Return the cooked vegetables back to the skillet that contains the shrimp.

- Add cherry tomatoes and lemon juice.
- Toss once again and finish with fresh basil.
- Serve and enjoy.

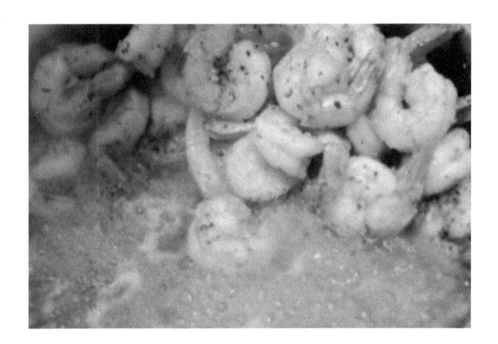

Mediterranean salmon kabobs

Ingredients

- 1 teaspoon of ground cumin
- 3 minced garlic cloves
- 1 zucchini, sliced into rounds
- 1 small red onion, cut into squares
- Kosher salt and pepper
- ½ teaspoon of ground coriander
- 1.5 lb. Salmon fillet, cut into cubes
- 1 lemon, zested, juiced
- 2 teaspoons of chopped fresh thyme leaves
- ¼ - ⅓ cup of extra virgin olive oil
- 2 teaspoons of dry oregano
- 1 teaspoon of mild chili pepper

Directions

- In a small bowl, begin by whisking together all the marinade ingredients of extra virgin olive oil, thyme, oregano, Aleppo pepper, lemon juice and zest, garlic, cumin, and coriander.
- In a large mixing bowl, put the salmon pieces, onions, and zucchini for seasoning with kosher salt and pepper. Do not forget to toss briefly.
- Carefully pour the marinade over the salmon and toss again to ensure total coating of the with the marinade.
- Leave to marinate for 15 – 20 minutes

- Thread the salmon and other ingredients typically onions and zucchini by the use of skewers.
- Arrange and heat the outdoor grill
- Arrange salmon skewers on top and cover the grill.
- Grill salmon kabobs for 6 – 8 minutes keep covered till fish is completely opaque. Endeavor to turn over halfway when cooking.
- Serve when hot or at room temperature.
- Enjoy.

Greek chicken and potatoes

This recipe is quite best for a family with hidden secrets in the lemon garlic sauce. Marinade the chicken for some hours or alternatively you can prepare it directly without marinade, the taste will remain remarkably sweeter.

Ingredients

- 1 teaspoon of black pepper
- ¼ cup of extra virgin olive oil
- Salt
- ½ teaspoon of ground nutmeg
- 4 gold potatoes clean, cut into thin wedges
- 6 – 12 pitted quality Kalamata olive oil
- Fresh parsley, for garnish
- 1 lemon, sliced
- ¼ cup of lemon juice
- 1 cup of chicken broth
- 12 fresh garlic cloves, minced
- 1 medium yellow onion, halved and sliced
- 3 lb. of chicken pieces, bone in with the skin
- 1 ½ tablespoon of dried rosemary

Directions

- Preheat your oven ready to 350°.
- Pat chicken dry and season with salt
- Organize the potato wedges and onions in the bottom of a baking dish.

- Season with 1 teaspoon of black pepper and salt.
- Add the chicken pieces to the seasoned potato wedges.
- Make the lemon-garlic sauce.
- Whisk ¼ cup extra virgin olive oil with lemon juice together with minced garlic, rosemary, and nutmeg in a small bowl.
- Pour all over the chicken and potatoes evenly.
- Organize lemon slices on top.
- Pour chicken broth into the pan from one side. However, be mindful not to pour the broth on the chicken.
- Transfer to the preheated oven while uncovered for 45 minutes - 1 hour until tender at 165°.
- Add Kalamata together with olives when removed from heat source.
- You can garnish with some bit of fresh parsley accordingly.
- Serve and enjoy salads and tzatziki sauce.

Lightning Source UK Ltd.
Milton Keynes UK
UKHW020718270521
384465UK00005B/193